Clean Eating Cookbook
25 Recipes To Help You To Slim Down

Table of Contents

Introduction

Those simple recipes are specially made for people suffering from obesity. It is quite effective for anyone interested in melting stubborn fat because some experts are available for your help. Basic problem while following any diet is a selection of food items. It can be difficult for you to decide what to cook on a regular basis to strictly follow your diet goal.

This book is designed for your help so that you can enjoy delicious meals without disturbing your regular diet. The book has something unique for foodies, such as Chinese food, Indian food, Thai and Italian food. If you love to enjoy Pizzas, then don't worry because this book also has pizza recipes for you.

Indian food: Samosas and poppadoms are special things in Indian food, but these things are full of saturated fat and highly nourishing. It is good to try the chicken and tomato based curry, spinach and yogurt based vegetables to keep your diet in limits.

Chinese: Noodles and plain rice are important parts of Chinese food, but you have to keep an eye on your portion size. The food items with chicken breast, plain rice, vegetables, and tofu are good choice to satisfy your craving to eat Chinese food.

Thai food: You will surely like steamed rice, meat, fish and tofu along with vegetables. Typical Thai food is full of coconut cream and saturated fat to increase the nourishing value. This book has health Thai food items that are quite safe to enjoy during your diet.

Italian Food: Tomato and vegetable sauce along with lasagna and salad will be a good choice for you. It is highly recommended to include almost 2 teaspoons of olive oil in your diet. You can try olive oil dressing along with a healthy salad.

Finally, if you like pizza, it will be great to try recipes given in this book. It will be good to try the pizza with thin crust and basic topping to avoid unhealthy content. This book will help you to satisfy your craving with healthy food without disturbing your meal plans. A variety of healthy recipes can help you to maintain your slim shape.

Chapter 1 – Indian Weight Watchers Food

There are some dishes for lovers of Indian food, but these are healthy with low amount of saturated fat:

Recipe 01: Special Tikka Masala

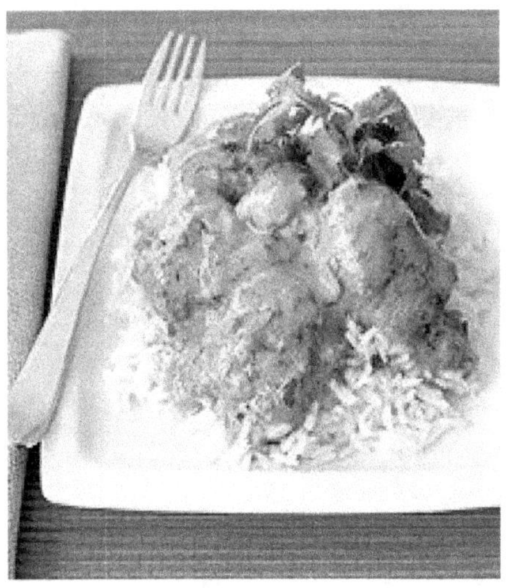

- 2/3 cup yogurt, low fat

- 1 teaspoon cumin seeds

- 1 teaspoon grated ginger

- 1 tablespoon lemon juice

- 2 cloves, powder

- 1/4 teaspoon black pepper

- 1 teaspoon cumin powder

- 1 pound chicken breast, without skin

- 1 garlic clove, chopped

- 2 teaspoons olive oil

- 1 teaspoon cumin seeds

- 1 small jalapeño pepper, chopped

- 8 oz tomato sauce

- 1/2 teaspoon paprika

- 1/4 cup cilantro, chopped

- 1 cup evaporated milk without fat

- 2 cups white rice, cooked

Directions:

Take a large bowl to prepare chicken and mix yogurt, lime juice, ginger paste, garlic paste, cumin seeds, cumin powder and black pepper. Now add chicken and mix all ingredients. Cover the bowl and keep it for 1 hour to 24 hours. Let one outdoor grill hot or use a nonstick pan.

Use metal or wooden skewers to skewer chicken pieces. Grill chicken pieces on a hot pan for 5 to 7 minutes. It will be good to soak wooden skewers in water for almost 30 minutes to avoid charring.

Meanwhile, make the sauce in a large and deep pan. Heat oil on a medium heat and add minced garlic and jalapeno. Cook them for one minute and now add paprika and remaining cumin. Now add tomato sauce and milk to cook on a low heat for five minutes. You have to mix frequently.

Now remove the chicken from the skewer and add into tomato mixture. Cook it for one minute and remove from heat. It is time to mix it with cilantro and serve with rice. You can enjoy 1 cup of chicken and ½ cup of rice in each serving.

Recipe 02: Saag Paneer (Spinach Cheese)

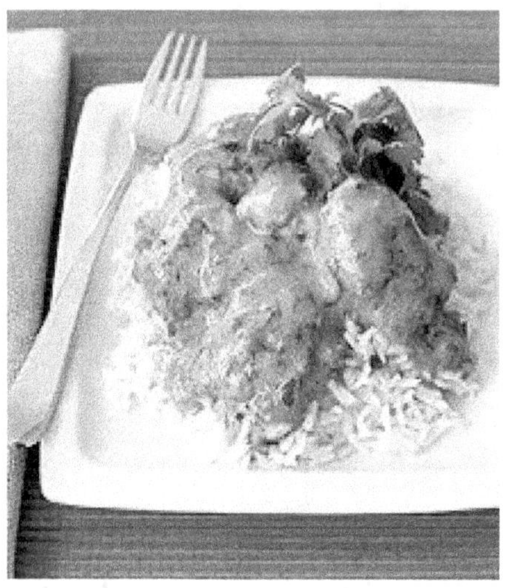

- 4 oz ricotta cheese (hard cheese)

- 1/2 cup onion, chopped

- 2 teaspoons olive oil

- 1 teaspoon grated ginger

- 1 teaspoon grated garlic

- 1 teaspoon cumin powder

- 1/2 teaspoon turmeric powder

- 2 garlic cloves, crushed

- 1/4 teaspoon table salt

- 10 oz chopped spinach, fresh

Directions:

Cut cheese to make cubes. Let one nonstick pan heat on a medium flame and add cheese to make them golden. It will take almost 1 minute and then remove cheese with a spatula and keep it aside.

Now add garlic, onion and ginger in the skillet to cook for 2 minutes. Put turmeric and cumin and mix together. It is time to add spinach leaves and cook for almost 2 minutes. Mix salt and return to cheese cubes. Cook it for one minute and serve with spinach leaves.

Recipe 03: Lamb Patties with Tomato and Peas

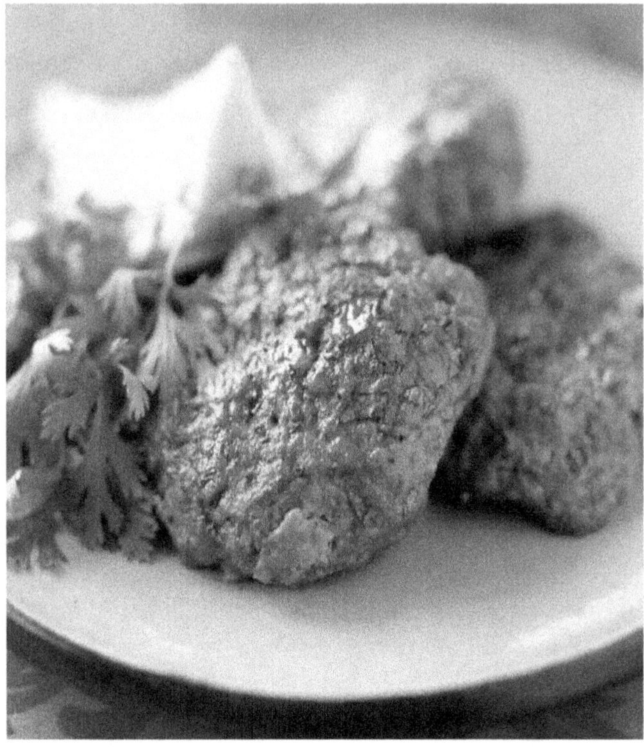

- 1 1/4 pound ground lamb, lean

- 2 teaspoon garam masala (mixture of spices, such as cumin, cardamom, coriander)

- 1 teaspoon cumin powder

- 2 teaspoons ground coriander

- 1/2 teaspoon turmeric powder

- 2 medium tomatoes, chopped

- 1 teaspoon sea salt

- 3/4 cup yogurt, low fat

- 1 cup green peas

- 2 tablespoons chopped cilantro

- 1 lemon, chopped into 4 wedges at the time of serving

- 1 teaspoon lemon zest

Directions:

Line a plastic wrap on the baking sheet.

Take a bowl and mix all ingredients except wedges of lemon. You can use your hands or a wooden spoon to mix all the ingredients thoroughly. You need to make almost 3-inch patties and keep them on baking sheet prepared in advance. Keep it in the refrigerator for 20 minutes.

Preheat a grill and cook patties on the grill or broiler. Slowly turn one side after 4 to 5 minutes. You can enjoy almost 3 patties in each serving with tomato sauce.

Recipe 04: Indian Curried Chickpeas

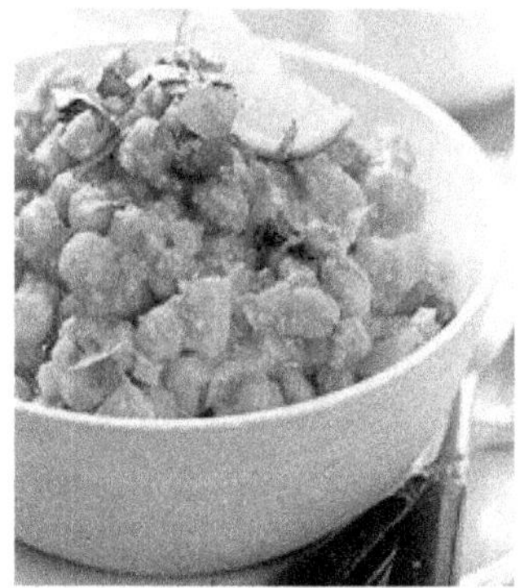

- 2 tablespoons dry coconut meat, unsweetened and shredded

- 1 jalapeño pepper, chopped after removing seeds

- 1 teaspoon coriander seeds

- 1 teaspoon table salt

- 2 Tablespoons filtered water

- 2 tomatoes, chopped without seeds

- 1 raw carrot, chopped

- 19 oz chickpeas, rinsed

- 1/2 teaspoon cinnamon powder

- 1/2 teaspoon cumin powder

- 1 Tablespoon cilantro, chopped

- 3 tablespoons yogurt without fat

Directions:

Add coriander seeds, jalapeno, coconut, water and salt in a blender to make a paste. Keep this paste aside.

Grease a nonstick pan and keep it on a medium heat. Now cook carrots, chickpeas and tomatoes to make them tender. Cook it for almost 10 minutes and then mix cinnamon, coconut mixture, yogurt and cumin to cook on a low heat for five minutes. In the last, sprinkle cilantro and enjoy 1 cup per serving.

Recipe 05: Delicious Spinach with Chicken

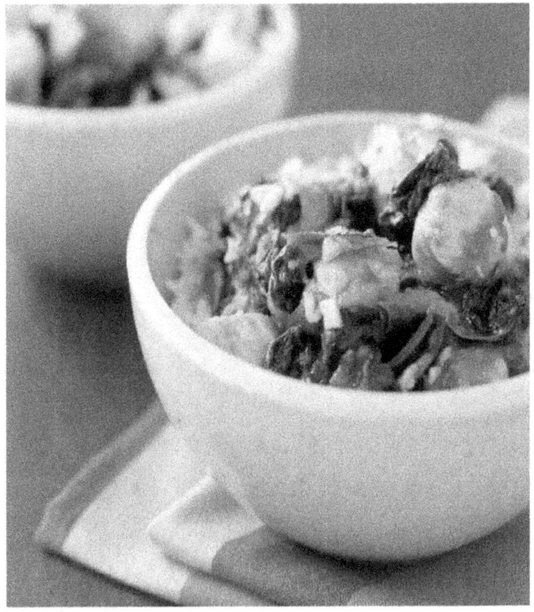

- 2 Tablespoons olive oil, (divided)

- 1 teaspoon coriander powder

- 4 teaspoons curry powder

- 1/2 teaspoons cumin powder

- 2 Tablespoons ginger, chopped

- 1 pound chicken breast, chopped

- 2 chopped garlic cloves

- 2 fresh tomatoes, chopped

- 1/2 teaspoons sea salt

- 10 oz. spinach, fresh leaves

- 1/4 cup water

- 2 Tablespoons cilantro, chopped

Directions:

Take a large nonstick pan and add 1 teaspoon of oil, coriander, curry powder, ginger, garlic and cumin seeds. Cook them on a medium heat and mix occasionally. Let them cook for 2 to 3 minutes to toast them. Now add the remaining oil and chicken to the pan and mix them well.

Now add tomatoes in the pan and cover it for 10 minutes. It is time to mix all the ingredients and add spinach to cook for 5 minutes. Keep it uncovered and mix well to combine. It is time for water and salt along with cilantro to add to the pan. Cook for 1 minute and enjoy 1.5 heaping cups in each serving. You can enjoy it with plain brown rice cooked with onion and bay leaves.

Chapter 2 – Chinese Weight Watchers Recipes

If you love to eat Chinese food, you can enjoy these recipes during your diet.
These are healthy for you!

Recipe 06: Lemon Chicken and Broccoli

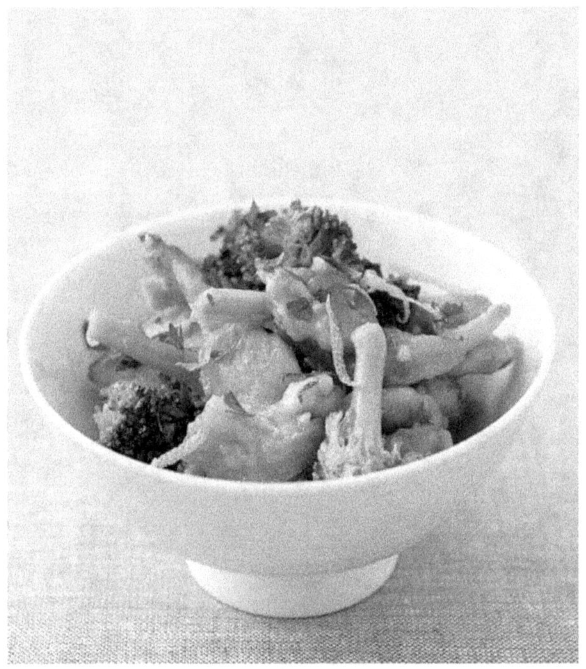

- 2 Tablespoons flour (all-purpose)

- 1/4 teaspoons black pepper powder

- 12 oz chicken breast(s), chopped

- 1/2 teaspoons table salt, (divided)

- 2 teaspoons olive oil

- 1 1/2 cups chicken broth, (divided, without salt and fat)

- 2 1/2 cups raw broccoli, take small floret

- 2 teaspoons garlic paste

- 2 teaspoons lemon zest as per taste

- 1 Tablespoons lemon juice

- 2 Tablespoons chopped parsley

Directions:

Mix 1.5 tablespoons flour, salt and pepper (1/4 teaspoons) and chicken in a bowl.

Take a nonstick pan and pour oil to keep it on a medium heat. It is time to add chicken and cook for five minutes to make it light brown. Now remove it in the plate.

Now cook 1 cup broth along with garlic paste in the pan. Let it boil on a high heat and use a wooden spoon to scrape the brown bits from the bottom. Now add the broccoli and cook for one minute.

Take a small cup and mix ½ tablespoon flour, remaining broth and ¼ teaspoon salt. Now add to the skillet and let it cook on the low heat. Cover it and cook to make a thick sauce and let the broccoli soft. It will take almost 1.5minutes. Mix chicken and lemon zest while heating.

Remove pan from the heat and mix parsley and lime juice; mix well. Its serving size is one cup.

Recipe 07: Bok Choy and Sesame Seeds

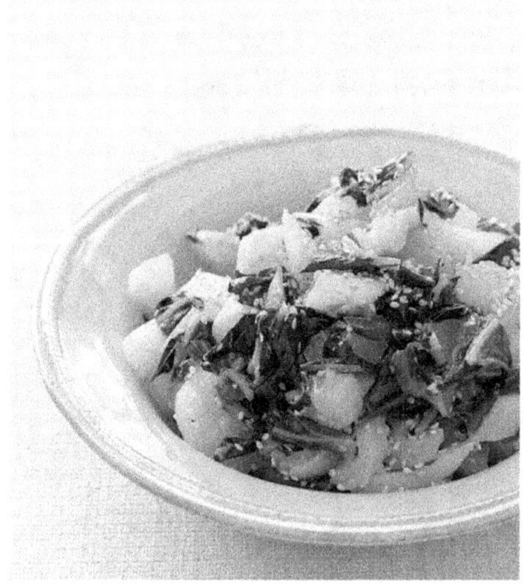

- 2 teaspoons canola oil

- 2 Tablespoons raw sesame seeds

- 1 Tablespoons ginger paste

- 2 teaspoons garlic paste

- 3/4 teaspoons salt

- 6 cups raw bok choy, chopped crosswise

- 1/4 teaspoons black pepper powder

Directions:

Take a large nonstick pan and keep it on a medium heat. Now add sesame seeds and cook to toast it lightly and mix frequently for almost 2 to 3 minutes. Now transfer these seeds to a shallow dish and keep it aside.

Use the same skillet and keep oil on the medium heat. Now add garlic and ginger to cook for almost 1 minute. It is time to add bok choy, pepper, and salt to cook on a medium heat for 5 minutes. Now sprinkle seeds and mix them well. Transfer to a bowl and enjoy 2/3 cup per serving. You can add red pepper flakes to make it spicy.

Recipe 08: Fried Shrimp with Snow Peas

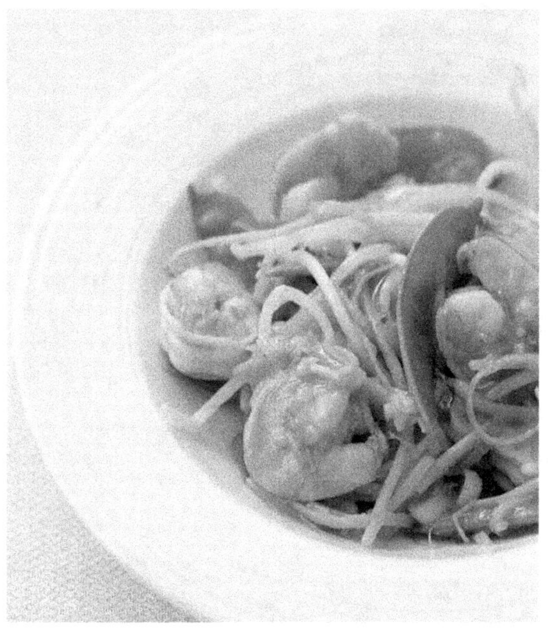

- 1 cooking spray

- 1 tablespoon ginger paste

- 4 medium raw scallions, chopped

- 1 tablespoon orange zest, crushed

- 2 garlic cloves, paste

- 8 oz raw shrimp

- 3 cups snow peas

- 1/2 cup orange juice, fresh

- 2 cups raw bean sprouts

- 1.5 teaspoons honey

- 2 Tablespoons soy sauce, low salt

- 1.5 Tablespoons rice vinegar

- 1.5 teaspoon cornstarch

- 1 teaspoon sesame oil, toasted

Directions:

Coat a nonstick pan with cooking spray and let it smoke on a high heat for almost two minutes. Now cook ginger, orange zest, scallions and garlic in this pan for 30 seconds.

Now add peas and continue cooking for almost two minutes. It is time to cook shrimp for almost 2 minutes. It is time to add soy sauce, orange juice, sprouts, and honey. Mix it and let it bubble for almost 1 minute. Now mix rice vinegar and cornstarch in a small bowl. Add this mixture to the pan and cook to make the sauce a thick but. It will take 30 seconds. Now transfer into a dish and enjoy 1.5 cups in each serving.

Recipe 09: Ginger Cod Fillets

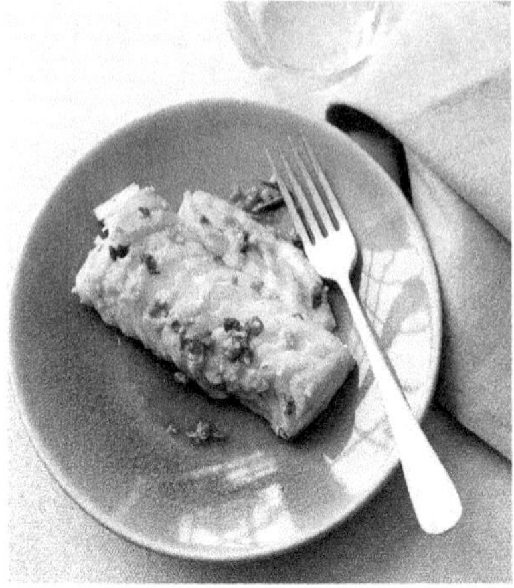

- 2 raw scallions, crushed

- 1 Tablespoon ginger paste

- 2 teaspoons garlic paste

- 1 Tablespoon sherry cooking wine (nonalcoholic)

- 1 Tablespoon soy sauce

- 1.5 pounds raw Pacific cod

Directions:

Keep the fish in a baking dish. Take a small bowl and mix ginger, scallions, garlic, sherry and soy sauce to pour over the fish. Let it marinate for almost 2 hours.

Take a saucepan and fill it with water to keep on a high heat. Let it boil and keep fish in a steamer basket. Now discard marinade and keep the steamer basket in the saucepan. The basket should sit above water.

Steam fish after covering the saucepan and wait for its complete cooking. It should be easy to flake with a fork. It will take almost 10 minutes. Divide into pieces and enjoy.

Recipe 10: Fried Rice with Eggs

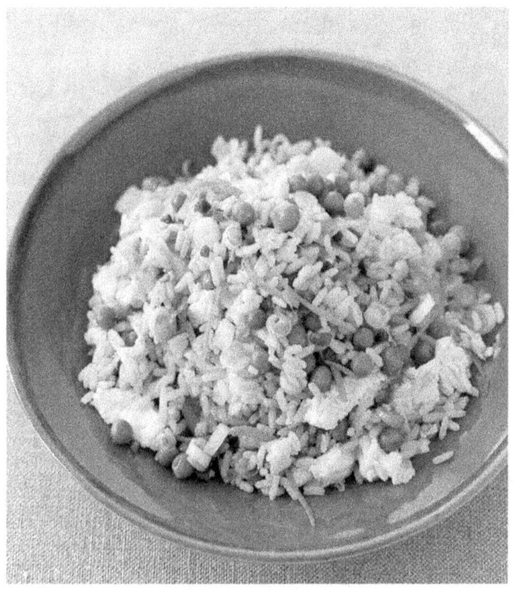

- 2 large eggs, beaten

- 2 cooking spray

- 1 cup raw carrot, ragged

- 3 cups cooked brown rice

- 1 cup raw scallion, chopped

- 1/2 cup green peas

- 1/4 cup soy sauce, low salt

Directions:

Use cooking spray to grease a large nonstick pan and keep it on a medium heat. Spread eggs on the bottom to let the eggs set. Now divide them into pieces with a wooden spoon for one minute. Remove eggs from pan and keep them aside.

Use the same cooking pan and keep it on the medium heat. Now add carrots and scallions almost 2 tablespoons. Cook it for 2 to 3 minutes.

It is time to mix rice, soy sauce, and peas. Wait, until it is heated through and mix twice for one minute. Now mix eggs and remaining scallions, cook to heat through. It is done and the ¾ cup is its one serving.

Chapter 3 – Special Thai Food for Weight Watchers

There are some recipes to satisfy the craving of Thai food lovers. These are full of healthy ingredients and perfect for healthy diet:

Recipe 11: Crock Pot Green Chicken

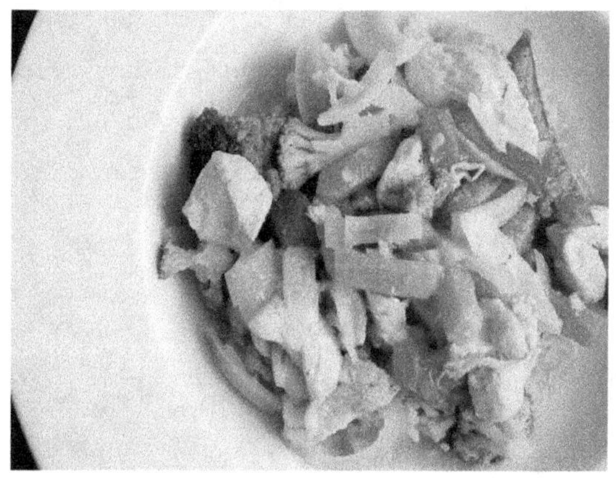

- 1 yellow onion, chopped

- 1lb chicken breasts, sliced

- 16oz vegetables of your choice

- 5 garlic cloves, crushed

- 15oz coconut milk, light

- Lemon juice, 1 lime

- 2 tablespoons brown sugar

- 3 tablespoons green curry paste

- 1 tablespoon cornstarch

- 1/2 teaspoon black pepper powder

- 1 teaspoon salt

Directions:

Put chicken, salt, and pepper in the crock pot and cover it with slices of onion. Take a medium bowl and mix lime juice, coconut milk, sugar, curry paste and add in chicken in the crock pot.

It will take 4 to 5 hours to cook. You can add vegetables in the last 45 minutes of cooking. Take a small bowl to mix cornstarch and 1 tablespoon of water. Add it to the crock pot along with vegetables and let it heat to make curry sauce thick. One serving is 2 cups.

Recipe 12: Grilled Chicken Breasts

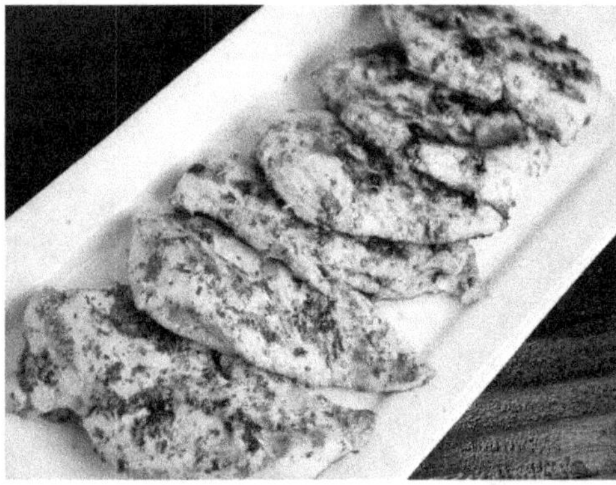

- 1.5 lbs chicken breasts, 6 fillets (no skin and bone)

- 1 tablespoons sesame oil

- 1 cup cilantro

- 2 tablespoons soy sauce, low sodium

- Juice from 1 lime

- 6 garlic cloves

- 1/2 cup chicken broth, fat-free

- 1 teaspoon salt

- 1/2 teaspoon black pepper powder

Directions:

Process all ingredients except chicken in the food processor to make them smooth. Now keep the chicken in a large bowl and pour blended mixture over the chicken. It should cover all the chicken and now keep it in the refrigerator for almost 3 hours.

Prepare a grill and cook it until the temperature reaches 165F, use a meat thermometer. Keep the breasts on the grill for 5 minutes before enjoying it. Your one serving size will be one chicken breast.

Recipe 13: Special Tom Kha Gai Soup

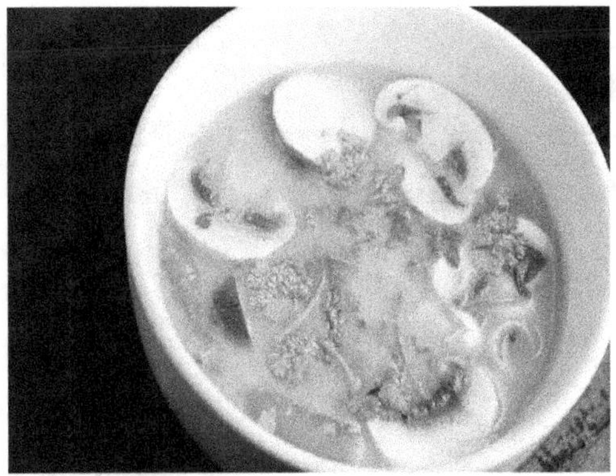

- 14 oz coconut milk, light

- 5 cups chicken broth, fat-free

- 1 tablespoon ginger, crushed

- 4 tablespoons fish sauce

- 1/4 cup lemongrass, chopped

- 2 tablespoons sauce (Siracha)

- Two limes, juice

- 2 tablespoons sugar

- 1/4 cup chopped scallions

- 1 cup peas, (sugar snap)

- 1/4 cup chopped cilantro

- 1/2 cup broccoli florets

- 2 zucchini, diced

- 1/3 cup carrots, sliced

- 1 cup mushrooms, chopped

Directions:

Take a large pot and add lemon grass, ginger and stock to let it boil. Keep it on a medium heat and cook for 30 minutes. Wait for lemongrass to release yummy flavors. Now add the lime juice, milk, both sauces, and sugar. Cook it for almost 10 minutes.

Meanwhile, blanch zucchini, broccoli and carrots in boiling water for almost 2 minutes. You have to make them soft a bit. Now take 6 bowls and equally divide vegetables. Distribute soups equally into each bowl with the vegetables. Serve with cilantro as a topping.

Recipe 14: Special Thai Chicken in Lettuce

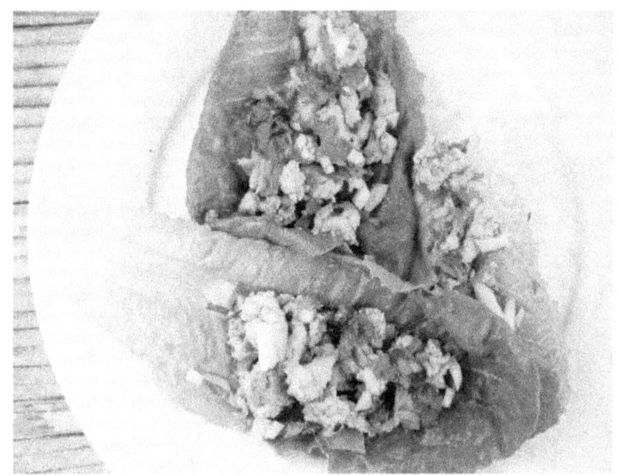

- 2 lbs chicken breast, ground

- 1 tablespoon olive oil

- 12 romaine lettuce, leaves

- 1 chopped onion

- 1 tablespoons sesame oil

- 1.5 tablespoons grated ginger

- 4 cloves garlic, crushed

- 2 tablespoons soy sauce

- 3 tablespoons fish sauce

- 2 tablespoons honey

- 1/2 cup chopped cilantro

- 2 limes, juice

- 1 tablespoons Thai chili, paste

- Salt and pepper

Directions:

Wash leaves and keeps on a paper towel. Take a large pan, heat olive oil on medium heat. Now cook onions and ginger for almost 3 minutes. The garlic may take another minute.

Now add chicken and cook with a wooden spoon. Mix sesame oil, soy sauce, lime zest, fish sauce and honey along with chili paste. Let it fully cooked and then keep on a low heat for another 7 minutes. Sprinkle pepper and salt as per taste.

Divide this mixture into lettuce cups and garnish with cilantro.

Recipe 15: Thai Cucumber Salad

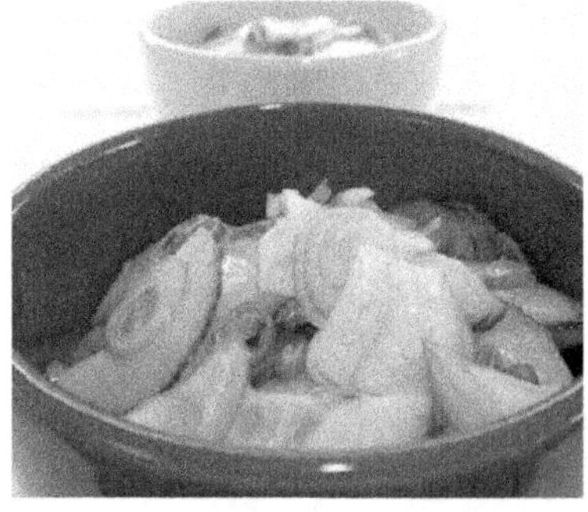

- 6 cucumbers, thin slices

- 1/2 cup water

- 1/2 cup vinegar

- 1/2 cup Splenda

- 1/4 cup shallots, thin slices

- 1 teaspoon salt

- 1/4 cup chopped onion

- 2 tablespoons green chilies

Directions:

You can use cucumber with or without skin. Mix water, vinegar, salt and Splenda to let the salt dissolve on medium heat and let it boil. Now remove from heat and let it cool at a room temperature.

Take a large bowl to combine all other ingredients and add vinegar mixture and enjoy.

Chapter 4 – Italian Recipes for Healthy Diet

There are some Italian recipes for weight watchers to add additional taste in your meals and avoid boredom.

Recipe 16: Italian Pot Roast in Slow Cooker

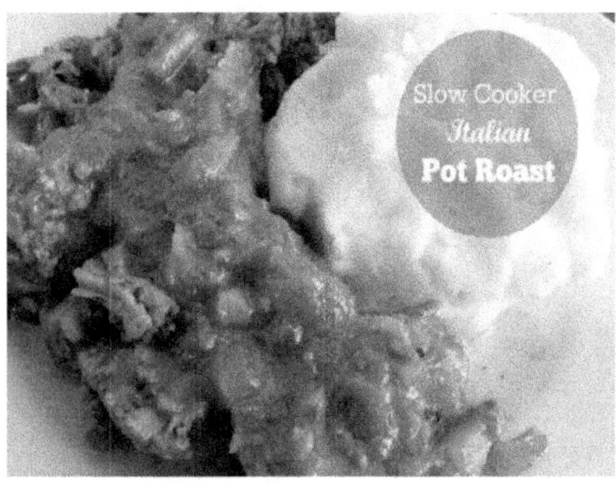

- 2 teaspoons salt

- 1 teaspoon black pepper powder

- 4 cloves garlic

- 4 lbs Eye Round Roast

- 2 teaspoons olive oil

- 4 chopped carrots

- 2 chopped celery stalks

- 1 cup chopped onions

- 1 cup red wine

- 2 teaspoons rosemary

- 28 ounces chopped tomatoes

- 1 cup beef broth, low salt

Directions:

Rub garlic, pepper and salt on the roast and keep it aside. Take a nonstick pan and heat oil on a medium flame. Now add roast and let it brown for 2 to 4 minutes. Now add celery, onion, rosemary and carrot in the pan to cook it for seven minutes.

Mix tomatoes and wine, and use a wooden spoon to scrape the brown bits. Now add beef broth and mixture of tomato. You can cook it on low setting for 7 to 8 hours. Take out the meat from slow cooker on a platter and cover it with aluminum foil.

If you want thick and concentrated sauce, transfer it to the saucepan and let it boil on a medium heat for 10 to 15 minutes. Remove off accumulated fat from the top.

Recipe 17: Thai Eggplant

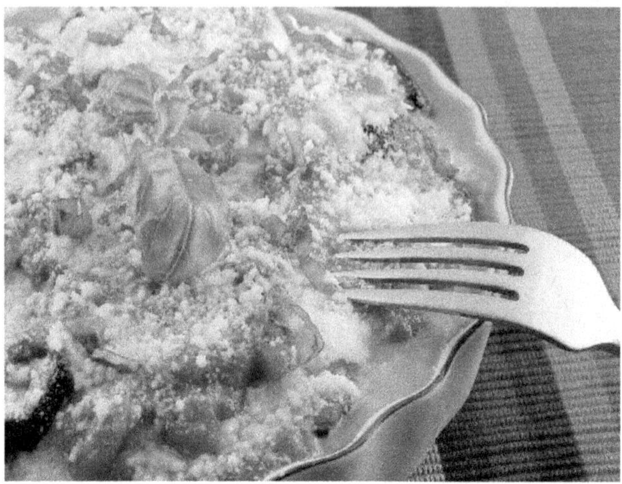

- 1⁄3 cup Italian crumbs (bread crumbs)

- 1 cooking spray

- 1 tablespoon grated cheese

- 1 tablespoon Italian seasoning

- 1 raw eggplant

- 1⁄4 teaspoon garlic powder

- 2 large egg white, (beat lightly)

- 1⁄2 cup mozzarella cheese, tattered

- 1 1⁄2 cup tomato sauce

Directions:

Prepare your oven at 350°F and grease a baking dish with spray. Set aside.

Mix cheese, seasoning, garlic powder and bread crumbs in a bowl and keep aside. Remove the skin of eggplants and cut off ends. Cut slices of eggplant and dip them in egg white one by one, then mix in bread crumbs. You have to bake these slices on a cooking sheet for almost 20 to 25 minutes.

Flip once while cooking and keep the layer of these slices in the bottom of baking dish. Now add 1/3rd of tomato sauce and cheese on the top. Repeat two more layers and bake until cheese is melted, and once again bake for 10 to 15 minutes more. Cut into pieces and serve.

Recipe 18: Italian Baked Tomatoes

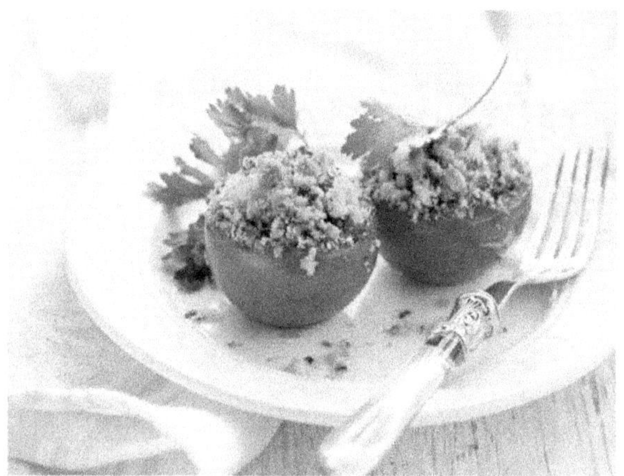

- 4 tomatoes

- 3 tablespoons bread crumbs, Italian seasoned

- 3 tablespoons grated cheese

Directions:

Preheat your oven to 350 degrees F or 175 C. Grease a nonstick cooking pan and set aside.

Slice tomatoes in half and remove its seeds and inner material. Now keep these slices in the prepared baking pan. Prepare a mixture of cheese and breadcrumbs in a bowl. Sprinkle this mixture evenly on tomatoes. Bake it for 35 to 45 minutes to make the topping brown. Serve with your favorite healthy sauce.

Recipe 19: Thai Chicken with Tomato Sauce

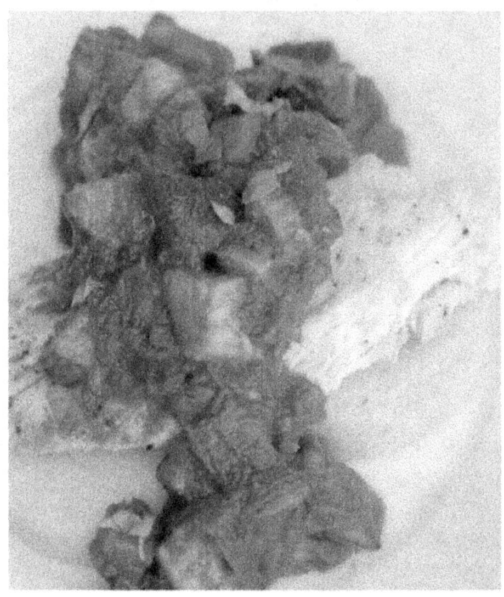

- 16 ounces plain polenta, 8 rounds (chopped)

- 4 chicken breasts (boneless, 5 oz each)

- 2 zucchini, chopped

- Salt and pepper as per taste

- 2 cups tomato basil sauce, low sugar

- ¼ cup water

Directions:

Heat a broiler in advance and grease a baking sheet with cooking spray. Arrange polenta in layers on the sheet and broil polenta for 6 to 8 minutes. Keep polenta at 4 inches distance from the heat.

Prepare a cooking pan with cooking spray and set it over a medium heat. Sprinkle salt and pepper on the chicken. Put chicken in the pan and cook it on medium heat for almost 10 minutes. The chicken should be lightly browned. Transfer to the plate and add zucchini to cook for 5 minutes. Add tomato sauce and water to cook for another 3 minutes.

Keep two slices of polenta on every plate. Top with chicken and sauce. You will prepare four plates.

Recipe 20: Italian Beef Stew

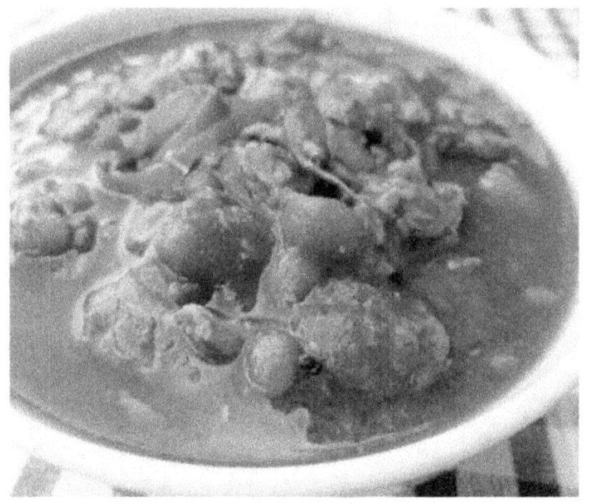

- 1 teaspoon salt

- ¼ teaspoon black pepper

- 1 pound beef, 1-inch chunks

- 1 cup onion, chopped

- 1 garlic clove, paste

- 14 - 15 ounces chopped tomatoes, undrained

- 1 teaspoon Italian seasoning, blend

- Tomato paste, 1 Tablespoon

- 4 cups beef broth

- ¾ cup lentils, rinsed

- 1 large zucchini, chopped

- ¼ cup basil

Directions:

Rub salt and sprinkle on the beef and add garlic, tomatoes, onion, lentils, beef broth and tomato paste along with beef in a slow cooker. Cover cooker to cook it on a low setting for 6 to 7 hours. In the last hour, add zucchini and let it cook. In the end, add basil and serve hot.

Chapter 5 – Special Diet Pizzas

Your love for pizza will not end because there are some special recipes to enjoy pizza during following a diet plan:

Recipe 21: Pizza with Grilled Mushroom

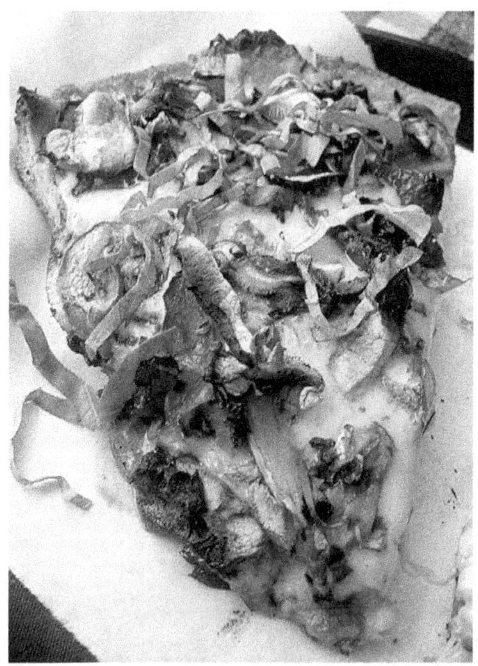

- 8 oz shiitake mushroom, remove stems and chopped

- 1 tablespoon olive oil

- 6 medium shallots, chopped after removing peels

- 1 cooking spray

- 1/4 teaspoon table salt

- 1/2 cup pizza sauce

- 4 whole wheat tortillas (medium)

- 1/8 lb provolone cheese

- 4 teaspoon grated cheese (Parmesan)

- 1 teaspoon oregano

Directions:

Prepare an oven at 450°F.

Take a large bowl and mix shallots, mushrooms, oil along with salt. Spread these things on a sheet pan and use cooking spray to coat them. Roast for 12 to 15 minutes to let the vegetables turn crispy and then remove from oven.

You can use a grill pan and keep it on a medium heat. Now spread 2 tablespoons of salt on every tortilla and sprinkle ¼ tsp oregano. Keep 1 slice of cheese on the top of each piece along with vegetable mixture and parmesan (1/4 teaspoon each).

Keep pizza on the grill pan and cook until edges become brown. It may take 3 to 4 minutes and now rotate pizza. Cook it until the cheese becomes bubbly and then leave it on the grill for 2 to 3 minutes more.

Recipe 22: Vegetable Pizza with Whole Wheat Crust

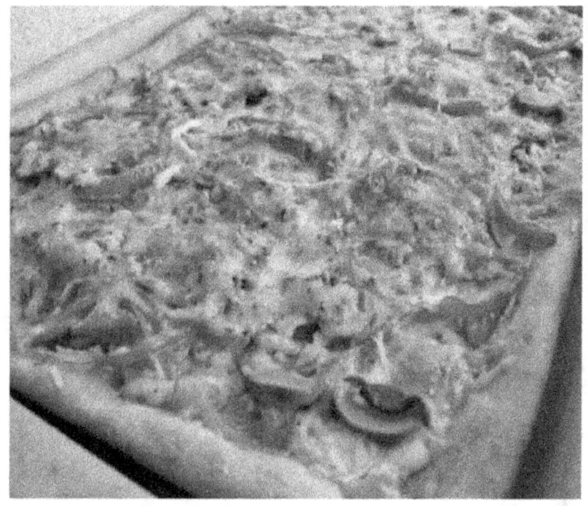

- 1 chopped onion, rings

- 1 pound pizza dough (whole wheat)

- 2 sliced tomatoes

- 1 cup sliced mushrooms

- 1 sliced bell pepper

- 2 pressed garlic cloves

- 1 teaspoon Seasoning Mix, Italian

- 1 cup mozzarella cheese, shredded

- 1 cup low-fat cheese, shredded

- ¼ cup Parmesan cheese, grated

Directions:

Prepare an oven to 400°F.

Now press the dough to fill a baking pan of 10 by 15 inches. You can use either stone or metal pan. Bake this crust for almost 7 minutes and remove from oven to keep on a wire rack.

You can add slices of pepper, tomatoes, onion and mushrooms on the crust. Press garlic on the warm crust and sprinkle cheeses evenly on the crust. Top with remaining vegetables, cheese and sprinkle Italian seasoning. Keep it in the oven and bake for 20 minutes to make the crust golden brown. Cut into 12 equal pieces with a pizza cutter or sharp knife.

Recipe 23: French Bread Special Pizza

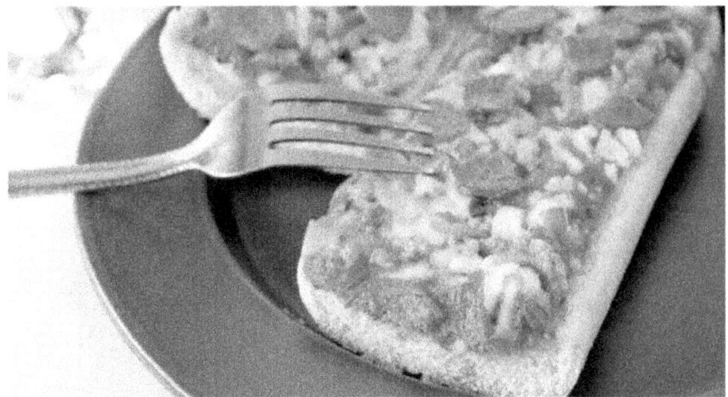

- Olive oil spray

- 3 ounces whole wheat baguette (it should be 5 to 6 inches long)

- ¼ cup bell pepper, sliced

- ¼ cup mushrooms, sliced

- ⅓ cup onion, ring slices

- ⅓ cup mozzarella cheese, low fat (shredded)

- ½ cup marinara sauce, low-fat

- Red pepper flakes

- Oregano

- 12 turkey pepperoni, slices

Directions:

Prepare an oven to 400 degrees.

Slice the baguette lengthwise and keep on a baking sheet with inside facing up. Now bake it for 5 to 7 minutes, toasted it lightly.

Meanwhile, lightly grease the non-stick pan and keep it on medium heat. Now cook onions, mushrooms and peppers to make it soft. It will take almost 5 minutes. Equally, distribute the marinara sauce and top each baguette, vegetable mixture, and the cheese. Now equally sprinkle pepper flakes and oregano on the baguette.

Now keep it in the pizza oven and bake to melt cheese and make bread crispy. It will take almost 5 to 8 minutes. Serve hot.

Recipe 24: Pizza Soup in Slow Cooker

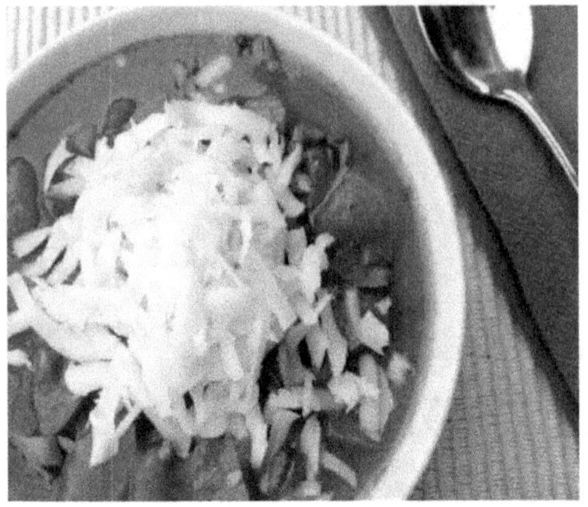

- 14.5 ounces chopped tomatoes

- 26 ounces marinara sauce, without fat

- 1 chopped onion

- 8 ounces chopped mushrooms

- 1 chopped pepper

- 6 turkey pepperoni, low-fat, chopped

- 1 yellow squash, chopped

- 1 cup water

- 1 tablespoon seasoning, Italian

- Low-fat mozzarella cheese, topping

- ½ cup dry macaroni

Directions:

Mix all the ingredients except pasta and cheese in the crock pot. Cover it and cook all the ingredients for 5 to 6 hours on a low setting to make vegetable tender. You should add pasta 30 minutes before serving and turn up it on high for 15 to 30 minutes.

Scoop into soup bowls and add the cheese at the top.

Recipe 25: Hawaiian Pizza Muffin

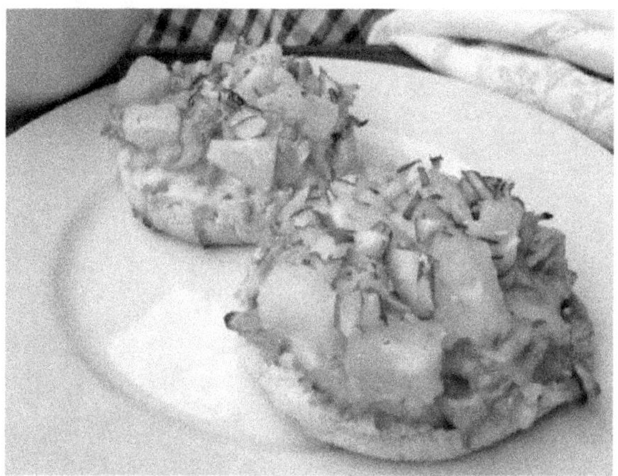

- 1 whole-wheat muffin, English muffin should be split in half

- 2 tablespoons mozzarella cheese, shredded

- 2 tablespoons sauce, marinara

- 2 slices beef, chopped

- 1 tablespoon chopped onion

- 2 tablespoons pineapple tidbits, drained

Directions:

Prepare an oven in advance to 350 degrees. Grease a baking pan with spray and foil.

Lightly toast the English muffin and remove from oven. Now spread 1 tablespoon sauce on each half of the muffin and keep muffin in the baking pan, distribute all ingredients evenly on each muffin and bake for 8 to 10 minutes.

Serve hot with your favorite low-fat sauce.

Conclusion

This is a successful plan to get rid of obesity and stubborn fat. This program can help you to reduce weight and you can constantly consult experts for your help. It is important to strictly follow the diet plan; otherwise, you will not be able to get desired results. This cookbook is designed to clear your confusion.

This book has Indian, Thai, Chinese and Italian recipes. These are healthy and so delicious that you can enjoy them without disturbing your diet plan. You can plan a menu for a whole month to save your time and buy all the ingredients at once from a grocery store.

If you are interested in reducing weight, you should try these recipes. This cookbook can be carried anywhere because the ingredients are easily available in every corner of the world. You should try these items at home.

If you want to throw a healthy party, 25 recipes in this book will make your work easy. You can prepare food that will entertain everyone. Your friends and relatives will surely praise your culinary skills. You can surprise all people with amazing mouthwatering recipes given in this book.